A DAUGHTER'S VOICE

on Caregiving for Her Parents

Roseline B. Woods

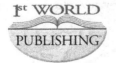

1st WORLD PUBLISHING

A DAUGHTER'S VOICE on Caregiving for Her Parents

Roseline B. Woods

Copyright © 2023 by Roseline B. Woods

Published by 1st World Publishing
P.O. Box 2211, Fairfield, Iowa 52556
tel: 641-209-5000 • fax: 866-440-5234
web: www.1stworldpublishing.com

First Edition

ISBN Softcover: 978-142183544-0
ISBN Hardcover: 978-1-4218-3545-7
LCCN: Library of Congress Cataloging-in-Publication Data

This material has been written and published for educational purposes to enhance one's well-being. In regard to health issues, the information is not intended as a substitute for appropriate care and advice from health professionals, nor does it equate to the assumption of medical or any other form of liability on the part of the publisher or author. The publisher and author shall have neither liability nor responsibility to any person or entity with respect to loss, damages, or injury claimed to be caused directly or indirectly by any information in this book.

Dedication

To my husband, Ron, for his love, devotion,
sacrifices and commitment.

Table of Contents

Acknowledgements

I want to thank my parents for their love and devotion with so little knowledge on how to raise ten children and doing the best they could. I thank them for passing on their talents – the nurturing and support from my mom, and the talents of storytelling, art and teaching from my dad.

Immense gratitude to my friend and counselor, Christine England, for many years of love, devotion, emotional support, and guidance in helping me build my confidence.

Special thanks to Christine Claudette Cote and Sharon Wright for the kindness and emotional support during each visit to help my parents.

I want to thank: My main editor, teacher and coach, Nancy Gibson, for her help and patience with me; MIU professor, Nynke Passi, for teaching and encouraging me about memoir writing, Rae Bird for teaching me healing free writing; My sister, Francoise, who shared her love of writing; My grownup children - Kevin, Melissa, Alia - and friends for having to listen to my babbling about my book.

Introduction

Let me take you on a journey of beauty, adventures, and inspiration through uplifting caregiving. I share my experiences of care and travel to make the journey of learning more pleasant. I fly from my home in the US to my parents' home in Canada to give help, support, and respite for my brother who is their main caregiver. As you will see, caregiving from the heart is similar in every country.

Through my stories, examples, and suggestions in this book, my intention is to offer you the knowledge to care for your loved ones in a more pleasant, easier, and more enjoyable way. I hope my stories will teach and inspire you to find ways to give the elderly respect and dignity for this unique time.

I've learned to use my heart and mind in making kind, fair, and loving decisions. My mother taught me: "to put myself in the other person's shoes." I imagine myself in the patients' situation. As their abilities decrease, I try to give them some control in their daily life by respecting their choices. This point of view empowers them to enjoy more peace, joy, serenity, and grace.

When we help make life happier for others, it makes our life better too.

Life is to enjoy!

This is a story of love, courage, humor, and creativity in finding ways to care for my parents when they needed more care, as their abilities are declining. This knowledge can also be used for any impaired person, young or old.

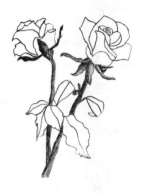

Chapter 1

Inspiration and breakthrough!

The trip home, 2012

My youngest brother Frank calls me to let me know that mom is coming out of the hospital. She has had a severe bladder infection. I worry that this might be the end. I get a flight from Iowa to Vancouver, Canada, and I decide that I want to be by her side for her last days.

I arrive in Vancouver on a clear, sunny day. From the plane I can see the whole city of Vancouver: the mountains with white peaks, vast ocean with the many small islands called the Gulf Islands sandwiched between the city of Vancouver and gigantic Vancouver Island. I'm overjoyed to be there again; it was my home for 14 years.

As I arrive at the airport, I see my younger brother Patrick who is there to pick me up. The next day Patrick and I leave for the long trip to Powell River. We arrive at the ferry terminal. A salty, fishy smell engulfs my senses, the brilliant sun blinds me, and the breeze blows my hair on my face. The sky is a bright, tender, baby blue like my dad's eyes. While waiting for the ferry to dock, I walk to the shore, pull my sandals off, dig my toes in the sand, and savor the coldness of the ocean on my feet.

I remember the first time I saw the ocean when we moved from Quebec by train to Vancouver, and then flew to Campbell River near my dad's work. My younger brothers Patrick, Frank and I lifted a few rocks and discovered tiny little scared crabs running away from us. The water was clear, pure, and salty.

Once on the ferry, we climb the stairs to the upper deck to the restaurant. I eat a vegie burger, some fries, and a Nanaimo bar for dessert (a layer of chocolate graham crackers with crushed almonds and coconut, then a sweet yellow mix of custard and frosting, and finally, a thick layer of hard chocolate on top). We visit the lounge, and I go on the outside deck. Looking around, I feel tiny beside the gigantic mountains, covered with cedars. The long, lacy branches of the cedars are like princess sleeves, above the rocky coves. Dried discarded logs are scattered on the sandy beaches, and the seagulls noisily beg for food.

Once off the ferry, for more than an hour we drive between the mountains and the ocean on narrow, winding roads that eventually take us to the next ferry. On this ferry in Earl Cove going to Saltry Bay, we watch multiple tugboats pulling logs to the paper mills and a few pleasure boats making waves. The tall evergreen cedars and the pointy firs cover the mountains. In the distance, I admire the mountain peaks, topped with snow all year around! With a bit of luck, one might be able to see a few Orca whales in the distance, but not today.

As I watch from the ferry, my thoughts drift back to memories of my mom. She cooked all the Christmas dinners until she was 79. She baked ten to fifteen pies: many meat pies (called Tourtières), a couple of raisin pies, a sugar pie or two (a creamy mixture of brown sugar, milk or cream and flour), and sometimes apple pies or blackberry pies. She always baked a turkey. On an ivory lace tablecloth, she displayed bowls of food: a massive mound of mashed potatoes, corn, and carrots. She tempted us with potato candies: cooked and cooled potatoes with lots of added powdered sugar, a little extract (either of vanilla, maple, or mint), rolled into a dough, spread flat and covered with a layer of peanut butter, then rolled up and cut into little candies. Mom often dyed the dough to make potato candy more attractive and inviting - red or green for Christmas, and blue, pink, or lilac for Easter. She sometimes bought or made a cake from our French tradition, "Buche de Noël", or Yule Log, which is a thin cake spread with jam, rolled up and topped with chocolate icing, and decorated with a holly leaf from our garden.

I remember my son Conner telling me: "I visited grandmama and grandpapa [my mom and dad] one day, and grandmama was sick. She couldn't get out of bed. I asked grandpapa, 'What is the matter with grandmama?' He told me that grandma was sick, but he was praying, and God was going to heal her. My son continued to tell me that he left, but came back later to check on her, and my dad was still praying! By his third visit, my son Conner said, "Grandpapa, God doesn't want us to be stupid; when somebody is sick, we take them to the doctor!"

Conner lifted my mom (who was more than two hundred pounds) in his arms, carried her to his truck, and rushed her to the emergency room. After examining her, the doctor told Conner that grandma was diabetic, and she had high cholesterol, which had caused a stroke. Her body was half-paralyzed on the left side, and she had lost her short-term memory from neglecting to bring her sooner. Had she come to the ER any later, she could have gone into a coma and died. Conner had saved his grandma's life!

I don't know what to expect as we approach my former home. My hands shake and heart pounds, after all, she is 92 years old.

I can see the old, gray, stucco house with round corners. I sigh as I look at the view from the driveway: the mountains of Vancouver Island, the ocean with ferries in the distance, the boat harbor with pleasure boats, sailboats, yachts, and fishing boats.

We climb out of the car. On the side of the driveway, I discover the lovely, sweet smelling, light-pink climbing roses that my dad planted for mom so many years ago. I pick three roses. I walk in and acknowledge mom sleeping on a hospital bed in the middle of the living room by the kitchen.

I notice the curtains are closed on the sliding glass doors past the foot of her bed. Where is the light and sun she used to love? On our phone calls, she would describe the ocean with the boats going by, the weather, and the sunset's display of colors: blue, yellow, orange, purple, and fuchsia pink. Her eyes are weak, and she can't handle strong light anymore.

She has lost so much weight. She looks fragile, delicate, and tiny in her white bed. Her breath is shallow. Her hair is short and white. She has only old, wrinkly, loose skin over thin bones like an old, wrinkled apple. Is this my lovely mom? I want to cry. My heart swells with pain to find her this way.

Frank has been the caregiver for several years now. He tells me that mom can't walk or talk anymore, and she sleeps most of the day. I don't know what to expect…Will she recognize us, Patrick and me?

I go closer to look at mom, and she wakes up. Patrick and Frank come to greet her, too. She opens her eyes with a questioning look, then smiles. I see liveliness in her eyes, her personality still shining through. I give her the roses; she smells them, touching them tenderly, and smiles.

The three of us are around her bed, and she slowly examines each one of us. She whispers, "My babies!" We are laughing, surprised that she is speaking, and that she recognizes us: the three youngest of her ten children.

Tears come to my eyes. I turn towards the kitchen, so as not to upset her, and wipe my face with a tissue. She takes my right hand and holds it tight. Patrick and Frank are now ordering Chinese food for dinner. They almost have to hand feed me, because Mom squeezes my right hand so tight, she won't let go of me. It is hard to eat with my left hand, but it doesn't matter. She is my mom, still alive.

In my suitcase, I bring out a short bed jacket and a matching beret I made for her with soft, fuzzy, fuchsia pink fabric. I show it to her, and her eyes widen with delight. I also brought a piece of blue silk fabric with pink and lilac-colored roses. I decide to put it over her white blanket to make her bed more cheerful. She smiles and surprises us by staying awake all evening.

Mom's Interaction with the Caregivers

The caregiver arrives for her night shift, and my mom has a mean look and won't cooperate. The schedule is twice a day, seven times a week. The first round is at eleven a.m., and the second in early evening between six or seven p.m. The job of the caregiver is to clean, bath, dress, feed mom and change her position on the bed: all that in 45 minutes to an hour.

As soon as mom sees the caregiver, her mood and body language changes; she tightens her eyes and hands, raises her fists, sometimes even tries to bite the caregiver. My brother tries to calm mom down by telling her he loves her and tenderly kissing her.

Mom wears diapers. She can't control her body anymore. Frank gently holds Mom down and restrains her hands to help the caregiver change her diaper and clean her. It breaks my heart to see them treat her that way. The caregiver reports in the daily notebook that my mom is violent again. It upsets me because my mom isn't a violent person by nature.

The only caregivers Mom cooperates with are the ladies that have some resemblance to the family, or friends of the family. When there is a friendly atmosphere of jokes and laughter, then my mom is more docile.

Mom eats little: a few bites of peach yogurt, or a little warm oatmeal, or sometimes cut strawberries, blueberries, or raspberries. She drinks a bit of coffee (mostly milk filled with vitamins). The caregiver helps her drink with a straw.

I detest seeing her so skinny, like my dad when he was close to passing. Two years ago, when dad died, she was quite chubby. That weight caused problems for her heart, and she became diabetic.

In her younger years, she had been hospitalized for thromboses three times, but she has survived it. In comparison, my dad rode his bicycle every day until he fell and broke his shoulder. He was in his eighties then. He kept himself healthier than mom, stayed slim and ate fewer sweets. Who would have believed that she'd outlive him? Yet now, she is getting near the end.

Mom Surprises Us

My sister Barb arrives from Sherbrooke, Quebec, our childhood home, two days after I have. She is coming to help us with mom. Mom hasn't seen her for a few years. Again, my mom surprises us by pulling the front of her gown down. She wants to show Barb that she had one breast removed from cancer a few years back. My brother describes her condition as senile, but she keeps on surprising us with her clarity and long-term memory.

The three of us try to help the caregiver today, but mom gets upset again. She puts up a fight and won't cooperate. Frank, Barb, and I put our thinking heads together: "If we were in her position, what would we want?" My mom had taught us to put ourselves in the other person's shoes and try to understand other people better. Now we have a decision to make: What can we do for Mom to keep her happier, more peaceful, and comfortable?

The first obvious thing is that she has no privacy; in the hospital, they have curtains around the bed. Barb suggests transforming unused sheets into curtains. Frank has two sets from mom's and dad's old queen bed that are still around the house. I chose the green, purple, and yellow one with big, bright flowers. Frank brings the sewing machine upstairs and puts it beside mom's bed. I sew the curtains, and she gets to watch me make them. I see her eyes following each move I make; so, I show and tell her what I am doing. She stays awake all afternoon. Frank has some nice wooden curtain rods that he installs on the ceiling around her bed. She now has privacy, with cheerful flowers. I hang the curtains and, voila, first step done to help mom feel better.

Mom's Special Spa Day

Next, we take care of her appearance, something to make her feel special. Barb and I discover that the caregivers are using a powdered stay-in shampoo. It leaves my mom's hair heavy, gummy, greasy, and flat. Barb is a hairdresser and has experience doing hair for the elderly.

She shows me a technique to wash a bed-ridden person's hair. She puts a small towel under mom's head to keep the pillow dry and raises the head rest, so mom is partly sitting up, just a bit. Barb sends me to the kitchen to prepare a basin of warm water and a little washcloth with a bit of baby shampoo. We wash mom's hair with the washcloth. I then clean the washcloth and rinse her hair with it until the shampoo comes out, and her hair is squeaky clean. We pat her hair with a small dry towel to take the water out. My mom falls peacefully asleep as she loves having her head touched and massaged.

My sister cuts her hair, and we dry it with the hairdryer on low as Barb styles it back away from her face. I continue by pampering her face with a small amount of coconut oil (coconut on warm days, olive or sesame oil for colder days, or almond oil for any day). My sister trims and cuts her "mustache" on each side of her mouth and pulls out a few hairs on her chin.

We continue by dressing her in a clean, flowery gown

and her new bed jacket I made to keep her warm and cheery. Mom points at the beret, then to her head, so we put the beret on her. We continue by putting lipstick on her lips. Mom points again to show us to apply it on her cheeks. I see her observing everything. She directs her hand to the beige makeup and points to her face, where she had scratched herself. We then camouflage it with the beige makeup. We show her the results in the mirror, and she smiles. We take pictures, and she looks as pretty as a porcelain doll. We are surprised that she manages to stay awake all this afternoon. We are having fun, and with that smile on her face, we know she is enjoying herself too!

Observing the Routine of the Caregivers

Barb and I consider the routine of the caregivers, thinking of how we would feel if we were in mom's place. My mom is often asleep, warm, and cozy under the blankets when the caregiver arrives. The caregiver first wakes mom up, pulls the blankets off, lifts up her nightgown, takes the diaper off, and starts cleaning her private parts. My mom tries to keep the blanket on, hold on to her diaper, and tries to hit, kick, or bite the caregiver.

The caregiver tries to feed my mom, but she is still mad and rejects the food. The caregiver cleans up the kitchen and writes in the daily notebook: how my mom is doing, what she ate, and whether she was violent, or just not cooperative. Then the caregiver leaves.

Knowing my mom had always been the boss of the

house, I'm thinking that this is what she would say, "How dare you come into my house, wake me up, pull off the blankets and make me cold, take off my diaper, and wash my private parts! You didn't ask me if I wanted you to do that? I don't feel ready. I'm still drowsy from waking up. I don't know if I feel hungry yet. What do you think you're doing without asking for my permission?"

Some Solutions

Barb, Frank, and I think it would be better if the caregiver would try this sequence instead:

1. Greet my mom and sit with her for a minute.
2. Make her a cup of coffee.
3. Feed her.
4. Clean the kitchen.
5. Clean and change my mom's diaper, bath her, dress her in her clean gown just before she leaves.

This routine works better for my mom because it gives her time to wake up slowly, stay warm, have her coffee, satisfy her hunger, and then she is ready to be cleaned. The idea is to give her time to adjust to a stranger, stay warm, and feel more respected in her own home.

Each week there are seven or eight different caregivers (with her short-term memory, they all seem like strangers). These caregivers come into her home and do things their way without considering what my mom wants. They are all well-meaning but seem to be trained more to get the job done -- FAST. Most of them don't think about what it feels like to be disabled. It's important to consider how my mom feels, and that it is her home they are in. (Being under pressure makes people forget that elders are still humans who feel and think.)

I have made friends with all the caregivers, so I don't feel restrained about talking with them. I explain that we want them to do things differently. The new sequence for my mom will help her feel better, be more cooperative, and hopefully happier.

An Example of More Successful Care Giving

Lea is one of the caregivers that comes several times a week. Sometimes she manages to rub lotion on my mom's body. The concern is that my mom can get bed blisters. I start to watch what she does. I notice that Lea does everything slowly. She is gentle and patient. She sits with my mom, tells her what she is going to do, gives my mom time to adjust, and observes her response. If mom responds well, then she massages her.

When I tell Lea our new plan, she is happy. She asks me to teach her some French so my mom can understand her. I tell her that my mom has hearing loss, and she doesn't always understand me either. Lea tells me she is a nurse but doesn't want to work in hospitals or nursing homes because she gets in trouble for taking her time with patients. The nurses are expected to clean many patients in an hour, but in home services the caregivers have 45 minutes to an hour to take care of each patient. Lea feels that it is fair and respectful to the patient to take more time. I notice Lea is more effective because of how she cares for my mom and handles each situation.

Breakthrough in Communicating with Mom

Lea and I are talking about how to communicate better with my mom. An idea comes to mind. I tell Lea that last year I came for my mom's birthday. My mom received many cards. I saw her read each card slowly and smile. I don't see Frank come in and he is listening to our conversation. I share my memory with Lea, "What if I write a note for my mom to see if she can still read?"

Frank looks enthusiastic, rushes out of the room, and comes back with a whole box of colored markers and a bunch of note cards. I write on one: «Voulez-vous une tasse de café?», and for the caregivers in smaller letters below, "Would you like a cup of coffee?" I put the card in front of her. I slowly adjust its position until I see her eyes moving from left to right. Her whole face lights up. She nods her head up and down in a "yes" gesture.

I send Lea to the kitchen to make a cup of coffee. I'm holding my mom's hand. She squeezes it tight, and I see big tears coming down her face. At that moment, I am ready to cry too. I realize that all this time no one had been asking her what she wants; no one knows how to communicate with her... I turn around and let a couple of tears come down my face. I wipe them off, turn back, and smile at mom as I don't want her to upset her. I kiss her tenderly on the cheek. Lea holds the coffee ready for her. I sit Mom up, and Lea helps her drink the coffee with a straw.

During the next few weeks, I write many more note cards: "I'm going to wash you now! —What would you like to eat? —Strawberries? —Yogurt? —Raspberries? — Oatmeal? —Ice cream? —Cake?"

Frank, Lea, and I sigh with relief and smile with satisfaction. We have had a breakthrough! We can communicate with Mom and all the caregivers can too, finally! Mom has a bit more control over her life which gives her dignity and power to have her desires fulfilled.

In the last couple of weeks of my stay, I train the caregivers to use the 15 cards I made to communicate with mom.

Nurturing Mom

Each day is different and special. My brother Clement comes for the weekend once a month. He sits with mom for a while, holds her hand, and shows her pictures of his family in an automatic battery-operated framed slideshow. Clement tells her who is in each photo, and when it was taken. Her face beams with delight. He leaves the pictures with Mom on her night table so she can watch them when she wants to.

Clement runs out of ideas of what to do with mom. Frank has been taking care of mom for ten years now because mom is afraid to go to a nursing home. When she was young, she saw old people being neglected and beaten in such places. Clement willingly takes on the job of taking Frank golfing or playing pool for a respite. Frank is always exhausted when I come to help and he needs a break. This is an immense help for Frank and me. I get to have Mom all to myself and Frank gets to take a break and have fun activities to enjoy!

Sometimes I leave Frank with mom, and I walk down to the beach for a break. I pick up beautiful rocks, seashells, pieces of wood, dried seaweed, or a couple of small dried-up crabs when I discover some. Whatever I can find to share with my mom, I bring it home. She touches the objects with delight.

I also bring her flowers almost every day from the garden dad had planted for her so many years ago: different varieties of roses, my mom's favorite. She smells and feels the delicate petals and her face lights up. I bring her the outside world that she can't visit herself. I put the flowers on her adjustable table, so she can enjoy them during the day.

On Easter Sunday, I bring her a string of tiny, decorative butterfly lights I found at the Dollar Store. I put them around the curtains, over her bed. If she wakes up in the middle of the night, she won't be in the dark. The string of lights serves as a night light, and creates a jolly, cheerful atmosphere!

My friend Claudia visits every Friday night while my brother plays poker with his friends. Tonight, Claudia brings a puzzle with colorful, magical fairies, and flowers. We spend the evening putting it together, and mom watches joyfully. We glue it together and put it up across on the opposite wall to Mom's bed beside the other photos.

Frank has mom and dad's wedding photo and a framed picture of Jesus on the wall across from her bed. She points at her wedding photo sometimes, and we bring it down to remind her of her love for dad. She nods "yes" and asks, "Where is dad?" Frank tells her that Dad is now with Jesus.

Frank's favorite way to enjoy a special time with my mom is to sit beside her and watch old-fashioned French and English movies, which have her favorite actors: Maurice Chevalier, Charlie Chaplin, Frank Sinatra, Fernandel, and others. They also love to watch old videos of French singers from mom's time: Edith Piaf, Charles Aznavour, Fernand Gignac, Ginette Reno.

Inspiration for This Book

The nurse practitioner comes for her monthly visit. She is surprised when my mom smiles and cooperates with the exam. The nurse practitioner turns toward me and says, "What did you do?" I tell her the story of the changes we have made as described previously. She is amazed and asks me if I can come to her monthly meeting to tell her staff what we have done.

She has never seen my mom so happy, friendly, and cooperative! I tell her that I only have a week before I leave. She asks me to exchange emails, and I promise I will let her know in advance when I am coming back.

I am so proud of what we did by acknowledging what my mom had taught us: "Put yourself in the other person's shoes!" With the help of Frank, Barb, and Lea, we have made these changes. We succeeded in making mom's life happier. We gave her back her power, her dignity, and her voice!

The next year, I come back but I can't go to the nurse practitioner's monthly meeting because she has a new boss who doesn't allow visitors. If she thinks what I have accomplished is special, then instead of a presentation, I can write a book about giving a voice for elders, and people with disabilities. By sharing my mom's story, I strive to inspire others to find a way to give their patients dignity, power, respect, and a voice when they have none.

Points to Remember

Caregivers

- Getting to know your patients is enjoyable and helps you connect and get more cooperation.
- Respect and treat them as you would want to be treated. My mom always told us, "Put yourself in the other person's shoes."
- Have a routine that is fair, respectful, and considerate to the elder:
  - o Acknowledge the elder when you come in.
  - o Give them time to wake up slowly.
  - o Keep them warm.
  - o Offer a beverage.
  - o Feed them.
  - o Give them water.
  - o Once they are fed and hydrated, they will cooperate in being changed and cleaned.
- Create a way to give the elder privacy while being washed and changed; it can be a curtain, a room divider, a separate room or just a shut door.
- It is important to take care of yourself and enjoy your surroundings to balance the difficulties that you are facing. Find the time to relax and focus on the positive to overcome the fatigue and discouragement that can set in.

Family & Friends
- Bring Interesting Objects:
  - Bring the world to them through sensory objects:
  - SIGHT: Books with large, beautiful pictures:
    - flowers, different countries, beaches, pottery, fancy dishes, dolls, chocolate, cars, or trucks
    - Videos
  - TOUCH:
    - rocks from the beach, colorful leaves, or assorted fabrics
  - HEARING:
    - Music, music box, eBooks, family recordings
  - SMELL:
    - Fresh flowers, soaps, essential oils, spices, perfumes
  - TASTE:
    - Snacks, fruit, juice, produce from your garden
- Story books to read:
  - Short inspiring stories about good deeds or whatever the person likes. Try: *Alice in Wonderland, Swiss Family Robinson, Paddington Bear*
- Enjoy fun activities together:
  - Puzzles, music, videos, card games, word puzzles
- Make Surroundings Cheerful:
  - pictures, quilts, Christmas lights, rocking

chair, photos with names and year beside each family member. Personal objects expressing who they are.

- Show and Tell:
  o Knitting, sewing, drawing, painting, sculpting, writing, gardening. If not possible to bring, then bring pictures of it.
- Bring music that they like, and maybe you like, too, and share this time together. Make it fun! Have a tea party and dress up! Give them the gift of joy!

Help Them with Personal Care

These things the caregivers may not have time to do:

- Make sure they have their personal toothbrush, brush, comb, shaver, and all personal necessities.
- Brush their teeth or clean their dentures.
- Brush their hair, shave, or pull-out unwanted body hair.
- Arrange to have their hair cut or styled regularly.
- Put their name on their clothing.
- If they are bed ridden, cut the back of shirt or gowns to make it easy to put on or take off.
- Supply enough pillows, soft personal blanket, shawl, or sweater.
- Pamper them with a massage: head, foot, hand, back or legs.
-

BE THEIR VOICE by helping them to be respected, empowered, loved, and cherished!

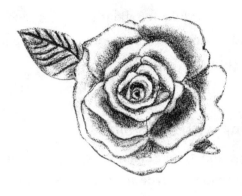

Chapter 2

The Dilemma of Arranging Care for My Parents

Beginning of the Caregiving Story, 2003

When my mom got out of the hospital after her stroke and was partly paralyzed, the ten children were concerned. Dad was slowing down, and mom had lost her short-term memory. She needed help walking, getting dressed, and going to the bathroom. She couldn't cook anymore because she would forget what she was doing.

Dad had never done much of the cooking. He was mostly making toast with peanut butter and jam. Dad had retired early from a back injury at his work in the logging camp. He had fallen off a boom and the metal cable had fallen on his back. With determination and strong will, he had managed to get stronger again. He could still ride his bike for about five miles each day; but he had to slow down because mom couldn't be left alone for an exceptionally long time.

Consulting with the Siblings

My siblings and I were talking, trying to figure it out. Our parents had not made any plans for their old age. All we knew was that they didn't want to go into a nursing home. This was the dilemma facing us.

My sister Barbara who lives in Sherbrooke, Quebec and I were talking on the phone about which of the siblings could take care of our parents. Clement and his wife Rena had a house in Nanaimo just a few hours away from our parents but were both working all day. Patrick had two children still in school and Frank lived in the Vancouver area in the city in a small apartment. I have been living in Fairfield, Iowa, for more than 20 years. The other siblings were not in any position to help with our parents much.

Years ago, with all the space I had in my house in Powell River, I always thought that I would have been the one taking care of our parents. When I mentioned that to Barbara, she said she was renting this beautiful white house in Sherbrooke with three bedrooms. One bedroom was hers; one was her hairdresser salon, and one was available for rent. She was looking for a new housemate.

Finding Secure Housing

What if she asked mom and dad to move in with her, back to Sherbrooke, Quebec? She said she would call them and ask if they wanted to move in. My parents accepted. They asked my brothers to get the house in Powell River cleaned and fixed up for sale.

That meant an airplane ride of over three thousand miles. With my mom in a wheelchair, they would need help from the airline.

It was a big change for both my mom and dad. With three of their children, sixteen grandchildren and all their relatives within two hours from Sherbrooke, Barbara thought she would get some help. Dad could walk to the mall four blocks away. Being in the French environment, dad would be able to talk to people more easily. For these reasons, it seemed the ideal situation.

Friction on the horizon

My parents had been used to having their own house. My dad liked carving wood to make gifts for the family like little wooden Santas with sleds, small reindeers, or tree ornaments. He was making a mess and had been used to my mom picking up after him.

He was born on a farm. He had always grown his own vegetables, raised his animals for food, fixed his own house, planted roses for my mom. He liked being busy, being outdoors and having his hands in dirt.

In contrast, Barbara had to keep her house orderly

and clean. After all she was running a business. People came in and out for haircuts, perms, hair coloring. She was busy. My dad thought that Barb's clients were visiting him as well. He would start conversations with them which would make them uncomfortable and late for their hair appointments. Barb decided to rent the basement suite as well as the main floor and moved all her hairdresser's equipment downstairs to have privacy. This made the cost of taking care of mom and dad much more. To make matters worse, my dad didn't like that she was a single woman and would go on dates sometimes. He started to think that she was having male company downstairs and that was why she moved the business there. Dad was from the old generation where people stayed married no matter what, and he wasn't shy to tell her what he thought. This was the last thing on her mind. The friction grew, and she couldn't go on like that. She realized that she had taken on a bigger job than she had expected. All this made her think she would have to put them in a nursing home soon.

Considering a Nursing Home

Our maternal grandparents had stayed in a nursing home a few blocks from Barbara's house. My grandparents had their own separate room with privacy. The residents entertained themselves playing card games, shooting pool, and participating in bingo in a large game room. The dining hall meant they didn't have to cook for themselves anymore and could enjoy other elders' company during meals. My grandparents were happy there. My mom had liked it then, but now with her memory lost, she wouldn't hear of staying in a nursing home.

My dad liked his freedom and would often walk to the mall. He almost got hit several times because he would forget to wait for cars when crossing the street. In the province of British Columbia, cars must stop if somebody puts their foot into the street; but in Quebec, the cars go fast and have the right of way. After over forty years of living in Powell River, B.C. he couldn't get used to the difference. It was a big worry for all of us, but especially for my sister who felt responsible.

Mom often wouldn't cooperate. She didn't like having to take a shower every day; but with incontinence, it was the best way to keep her clean and smelling good. My sister did her hair each day and mom looked beautiful. Barbara thought that she would get a lot of help from family members, but they were all busy with their own children, work, and the fast life in the city. Although everyone did what they could, it wasn't enough.

Barbara had taken on more than she could handle. She was getting to be very exhausted. She started looking into putting them in this same nursing home as my grandparents had been. My parents heard her talking about the nursing home and were very upset. They thought they couldn't trust her anymore.

Several Siblings Share the Load

During that year, the sawmill in Vancouver where my brother Frank was working shut down. He decided to go to Powell River and live in my parents' house and planned to fix it up and get it ready to sell. My parents' house had three bedrooms downstairs with a large hall with kitchenette and small washroom for family reunions. The upstairs had two more bedrooms, bathroom and kitchen connected to the living room with the most beautiful view of the ocean. The rooms in the house needed painting. The outside stucco needed patching up. The yard had a lot of junk to get rid of. The inside had a collection of useless objects. With all this work to do he was going to stay for a while. The large space gave him the option to get a roommate to share costs while he was fixing the house. My parents couldn't afford to pay for both places, so Frank was paying rent with his unemployment check.

Not long after Frank settled in, my dad called him and asked if he could take care of them in their own house. They were homesick. Frank agreed. He didn't have a job and being divorced with his daughter in college meant that he was free. He was the only one of all the siblings who was available and had the time.

Would Frank be able to last for the long stretch ahead? I decided to come once a year to give Frank a break so he would last. Clement lived in Nanaimo on Vancouver Island just a few hours away. He would come once a month to check on my parents.

Patrick decided to help me get to Powell River from

the Vancouver Airport. Patrick still had teens at home, but he would try to visit a few times a year as time would allow. All of us who could, volunteered to share the load. We would also give Frank moral support: calling him with words of encouragement and surprising him with short visits. Since my parents weren't wealthy, the government would pay for caregivers as needed. The biggest dilemma was resolved. Peace at last!

Points to Remember

What to do when your parents can't take care of themselves anymore?

Look for solutions.

Make a list of your parents' likes and dislikes with regards to their living space.

Talk with family members (or family substitutes) and with doctors, nurses, social workers, therapists.

Research and educate yourself about the following:

- their medical evaluation – physical, mental, emotional – their abilities and limitations
- availability of family or friends,
- social services – what they can provide
- elder resources – associations, organizations, community centers, churches
- their insurance – medical, life, disability, long-term care
- their finances – property, investments, retirement funds, pensions, social security
- their legal agreements – will, health care power of attorney, living wills

Effective communication and being well-informed is the key.

Check different options – assisted living, home care, live-in caregiver, or nursing home.

If a nursing home is the option of choice, then look at many different ones. Gather information about the different nursing homes and what they have to offer. Consider the following:

- Location - What is available in their area, or your area?
- Quality – the facility, the personnel, level of care needed.
- Cost
- Availability
- Limitations
- Contract

Compare options and decide on the best one. The first option may not work out, then try another one.

Be realistic with your decision and be good to yourself. After all we are all human and are not perfect and have limitations as to how much we can do. Please keep that in mind.

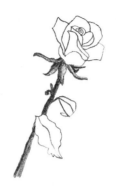

Chapter 3

Home Again

Home Again, 2004

My brothers, son, and nephew along with the Church group cleaned up the debris from the yard: old washing machines, lawn mowers, wooden planks, big pieces of plywood, tree branches, rusty tools, dried up cans of paints, and many other useless things sitting around and rusting. My dad collects junk and thinks he's going to fix it someday.

Powell River is like an island because the mountains circle it, making it impossible to drive to Vancouver. The recycling is expensive because of the extra cost of the ferry boats to discharge of it. Frank got rid of the unwanted clothes, boxes of unnecessary junk like old pots and pans, used books, bottles, jars, old magazines, ripped towels, broken cups and lots of odds and ends.

He replaced it with his own kitchenware: matching glasses, coffee cups, stainless steels pots and pans, set of ceramic dishes, dish towels, bath towels, new sheets, and pillowcases. He brought his vacuum cleaner, and all the cupboards are now organized and cleaned. Having an organized house will simplify the caregiving.

Frank and Patrick pick our parents up from the Vancouver Airport and welcome them with warm hugs. Mom and dad are overjoyed. They all visit Queen Victoria's Garden in Vancouver. They enjoy the colorful flowers and trees; daffodils, daisies, assorted rose bushes, cherry trees with blossoms, Japanese maples, flourishing dogwoods, and arbutus trees that lose their bark. The warmer weather, the beautiful sunny day gives them hope of better days. After all it is called the Sunshine Coast, isn't it?

Our parents are now in their own home secure with my brother Frank's help. Dad can ride his bike 5 miles a day, but mom can't be left alone for very long. Frank works for a moving company but comes home for lunch to feed mom and dad. Dad can hold mom's hand to take her to the bathroom, get her dressed each morning, and help with cleaning her up. Life is good and all the siblings are happy to know that our parents are looked after. Frank takes them to church every Sunday. Retired church members gather for a luncheon after church and also every Wednesday. These are the only outings mom and dad have.

I come to visit every year, and this year I feel sad for them and think that my brother has been lazy until I go to church on Sunday with mom, dad, and Frank. I find out that mom often discharges in her pants, and Frank spends a lot of time in the women's bathroom changing her diaper. After this I appreciate my brother for his courage and patience with no more judgements.

I cook big meals and find out that mom pushes the plate away refusing to eat. I am concern wondering what is wrong. Is she sick? I finally realized that mom's short-term memory won't let her eat anything unfamiliar, she only eats what she remembers. She likes French fries, burgers, chicken, potatoes, peanut butter on toast with strawberry jam, eggs, carrots and maybe some yellow beans. When any of us make toast for her she won't eat it unless we butter the toast to the edge with the peanut butter and jam. If not, she pushes it away. I think she is just being fussy and picky until I notice that her dentures are wearing out, so all the food needs to be soft. I guess it must hurt her gums when she chews.

On Valentine's Day I buy some big chocolate hearts for both mom and dad. Dad opens it up and takes little bites, and then I see mom put the whole chocolate in her mouth. It is sticking out because it is bigger than her mouth. The chocolate melts and falls on her clean clothes. Frank and I laugh because she wouldn't have done anything like that in her earlier years. Born in Sherbrooke, Mom was dressing elegantly with good manners and speaking a good artic-ulated French. Comparatively, my dad had a grade three education, speaks a slang French, dresses like a farmer, wears dirty boots in the house, soaks his bread to clean his plate and drinks the liquid from his bowl. Dad knows how to dress like a gentleman and use finer manners when going out but doesn't like it much. (Frank and I mention how the roles are reversed right now.)

A few days later it is dad's birthday. I make a spice cake and serve it with ice cream. Mom hasn't forgotten about cake and ice cream, and she eats it all. I give him his presents: a flytrap plant, a shoehorn, and a funny card about getting old. He reads the card but doesn't smile. Then I see that he doesn't think it is funny to grow old. Frank and I are eating our cake and chatting, then Frank runs to my dad's side. I see my dad with his finger in the plant as Frank pulls the plant away just in time. He says "No dad, you can get hurt. Don't put your finger in there."

Well, I think, *so much for that present but at least he liked the cake because he asked for a second piece.*

Frank says, "They are worse than children." I notice that the roles are changed now: we must parent them, yet they are adults.

We are laughing again. What can we do? We never know what to expect, or what they will do next? They are quite entertaining with surprises every time we introduce something new. We just need a sense of humor to survive all the different situations as their inhibitions are disappearing!

Twice a day the caregiver comes to help with my mom. Today Sophia comes in, but mom, for some reason, doesn't seem to like her. She is about 40 years old; she wears lots of thick makeup, red lipstick, drawn eyebrows, fake eye lashes, tinted hair. She has a bit of a theatrical look with a heavy European accent. She is bossy. She takes my mom to the bathroom to clean her. Mom is hesitant. She goes, but not happily. I hear my mom say something loudly but am not sure what she said. When Sophia comes to the kitchen to prepare the food, we ask her what is the matter? She says that she prepared a wet washcloth and wanted to encourage mom to stay independent. She told mom to wash her face.

Mom said, "YOU wash YOUR face!"

Frank and I laugh with Sofia. In my mom's time, the only women who wore makeup like that were either actors or ladies of the night. We acknowledge that it must be why mom reacted this way. Luckily, Sophia has a good sense of humor.

Later my dad falls while riding his bike; he breaks and dislocates his arm. Frank takes him to the emergency room, but he refuses to let them operate on him. He is afraid of dying during the operation. He is no longer able to help with mom, so Frank can't work anymore. Now Frank must take care of both mom and dad. Clement retires from his teaching job and comes every two weeks. The caregivers are scheduled for more time to help with my dad too. I still come once a year but stay longer, sometimes a month or two.

The next time I arrive to help, Frank is exhausted and depressed. Frank is a tall 6'1" and has a medium muscular chest. Today his curly hair is messy and a bit long, his face is pale and unshaved, and his dark brown eyes are streaked with red. Dark circles under his eyes beg for more sleep. Frank usually smiles, laughs, and jokes, but today he briefly greets me and runs out the door to work on his car.

That night he leaves me to sleep in the room next to our parents' and disappears downstairs to rest. I don't have time to recuperate from the long trip and I am suddenly in charge. The curtains are closed in the living room, dad has not been shaved; his shirt is dirty from dropping food when he eats. Mom is still chubbier, her hair is cut unevenly, and too short. I kiss her and she wants me to sit with her, so, I do. What a difference from last year when I came. Now the room is gray and cries with sadness.

Dad is happy to see me. With a pout, he shyly asks me to cut his hair and shave him. That takes me back to when I was nine years old, and my mom had her first thromboses and dad needed a haircut. Mom cut everybody's hair in the family, but she wasn't available. Dad asked me to cut his hair. I said, "No." Dad didn't take "no" for an answer. He told me to cut straight along the comb he was holding, and I did. Here I am so many years later and much more confident since I always cut my husband's hair and sometimes my own.

Dad is my hero, the man who sometimes defended me when my brothers were picking on me; the friend who helped his neighbors and extinguished fires before the firemen arrived; the beloved uncle who played cards after church every Sundays and loved maple walnut ice cream; the playful joker who told funny, slightly indecent stories, and made everybody laugh.

He liked to tell the story of his father: "My father lived across the lake on his beautiful farm. It was winter, everything was made of snow and ice. His wife was sick, so he took care of her first, but he was going to be late for church, which was across the lake. He wasn't sure if the lake was frozen enough, but he decided to take a chance since it would take much longer to go around. He got in the buggy with his horse going as fast as he could across the lake. When he arrived, the guys were waiting for him outside the church as usual. They asked him: 'How is your wife?' He was still nervous, shaken from the ride and hard of hearing. He thought that they were asking about the ice. He said, 'She was cracking and popping, but I got on her anyway.' His buddies burst out laughing and he didn't know why until one of them told him that they wanted to know how his wife was, but not the ice. "

That story made everybody laugh, and they teased my grandfather about it for the rest of his life. My dad heard the story when he was a young man and had fun telling it. I loved his side-way smile and mischievous eyes when he told a tale, and everyone loved him for it.

I get the old scissors and cut his thinned gray hair. Then dad takes out his metal razor with single-edged blade, his brush and soap; this must be done the old fashion way. He then shows me how to shave his aged, wrinkled face. His beautiful grayish blue eyes watch and guide me. He helps me by sticking his tongue in his cheek to stretch the old, dried skin on his face to make the job easier. I manage to shave without cutting him, and he kisses me on the cheek. What an honor to be helping dad.

His walk is slower these days, the arthritic in his body is worse, his back curves down, his bones are thinning as he must have osteoporosis, but he won't go to doctors. The pain he endures from his broken arm and torn muscles has stolen his mischievous smile I loved so much. I cherish each moment because who knows how long he still has?

Dad worries about mom. She won't take her pills for her heart and her diabetes. She hides them everywhere; we find them stashed in the couch, her pockets, some tissues, even floating in her glass of water. Dad gets mad at her, and I must calm him down. He is hard of hearing, so I write him a note saying that it is ok if she misses a few pills since Frank watches her diet. I reassure him that she won't die from it. Dad reads the note repeatedly, which gives him peace.

That next day the caregiver Sophia comes to help dad with his bath for the first time. Like my mom, dad is not comfortable with her, since for him she represents a loose lady with all that makeup she wears. When she takes him to the bathroom, he stops her and tells her that he has never slept with anybody but my mom and that she is better to be careful how she handles the washing. She thinks it is funny and tells us about it. Life was so different in my parents' generation.

Nourishing the Heart

The next year when I come to help, my mom has very long nails and won't let anybody cut them. She hurts my dad when she wants to cuddle, and he gets mad. She won't let me, or Frank, cut them, and not even Clement when he comes to visit. We are wondering why she is refusing. I call my beautician friend Claudia who will visit me tonight, and I talk to her about it. I know that mom likes nail polish, so I ask if she can bring some. Claudia arrives showing mom three different color of nail polish: pink, lilac and red. She chooses the red one and offers her hands ready for her to do her nails. Claudia and I have fun making her pretty. She loves her red nails and shows everyone. All she wanted was to feel pretty but couldn't express herself. The problem is solved, and everyone is happy!

Every Friday night while Frank has his friends over to play poker downstairs in the big recreation room, Claudia comes to visit mom, dad, and me. This week she brings her little mini white poodle, Bebe, to spend time with us. Mom and dad love the change of pace and adore the little female dog. They take turns holding her and petting her. Mom holds her too tight sometimes and we must help soften up the embrace, but Bebe let's her know with a sharp bark. We have fun holding Bebe while watching a movie, but mom gets jealous. We just can't reason with a dementia patient; mom can't understand; she often just lives in her own little world. When my babies were little, I would lose a sense of reality sometimes from not going out enough, especially when they were sick, so I can relate to mom a bit.

This next week Claudia brings a small machine vibrator that we put at mom's feet. This machine is made for people that are not exercising enough to help improve circulation in the whole body. Mom and dad try it and they enjoy it as they ask for their turn again and again. I hope that it will help their health. I want them to experience more joy in life. Claudia is a wonderful, knowledgeable friend. I cherish my times with her; she's helpful and a valuable friend.

Frank Takes a Mini Vacation!

Frank takes off to go to Vancouver for the weekend to see Patrick and have some fun.

I'm alone with mom and dad. A list of people to call in case of an emergency hangs on the kitchen cabinet. I also have Frank's cellphone number and Patrick's, so everything should be fine.

I keep the cooking to simple food they know since they don't have the flexibility to try things that are new, especially mom. Mom and dad are watching tv but occasionally mom says a remark unrelated to what is going on. I find the remarks strange, and she seems not to understand any of what is happening. I switch the channel to old movies or music, which they can relate to better. The new fast-paced life seems too much for them to understand. Their brains have slowed down a lot in their old age. Everything must be presented slowly and clearly.

I keep on seeing mom press her hand on her heart and

after a few times I keep a close eye on her. I start to get worried that she's having a stroke, so I try the emergency phone numbers to get some advice from his friends. Then I try my brothers' cell phones, but nobody answers. I talked to a nurse at the hospital, and she recommends I call 911. I dial 911, but they say they must come over to decide. When they arrive, they want to take her to the hospital to be checked. I don't want to upset her, but that is the rule in the province of British Columbia. I let them take her in. Dad and I follow the ambulance with the car. The doctor checks mom and she is fine. Her heart rate is perfect, but dad is very upset.

We go home and dad keeps on saying, "We almost lost mom."

I try to reassure him, but he doesn't understand and keeps on saying: "Yea, we almost lost her today."

He looks sad and distressed. Frank gets my message and calls back, and I tell him what happened. He is upset because he says that dad will be difficult and depressed for at least a month or two. I apologize and explain that nobody was reassuring me or helping me. What was I supposed to do? Seeing them only once a year makes it difficult to judge a situation.

For several days, my dad sits on the couch with his head down. When I pass by, he reaches for my hand and squeezes it saying, "We almost lost her." Each time I reassure him.

On Sunday, a friend from their church helps me with dressing and getting them into the car to go to church. I sit between them in church and enjoy the joyful singing. I grew up going to the Roman Catholic school and church. My parents switched churches in their old age because they wanted to read the Bible and make their own interpretation. It makes sense to me, but I miss the old traditions of my dad blessing us, his children, once a year. That has been replaced with lots of beautiful uplifting songs. I like it, but it is so very different.

After the service, I go through the drive through at McDonald's and buy them chicken sandwiches and fries. I continue my route to Wellington Beach and park on the hill. I encourage them to admire the view of the boats going by and people having a picnic on the sandy beach as they eat their lunch. I don't open the doors to let them out, since I'm not strong enough to help them in and out of the car.

My thoughts go to my dad who in 1969 moved ahead of the family to British Columbia from Quebec to join my cousin for work. Dad was working in a logging camp putting together the booms (after being cut, the logs are rolled down to the ocean, the workers drill holes in the end of the logs and put large metal cables to tie them together into what is called a boom) to be pulled to the Paper Mills by tugboats.

Nine months later the twelve of us travelled together and arrived on August 1, 1970: my mom, my sister with her husband and five children, plus my brothers Clement, and two younger ones Patrick and Frank. Dad had borrowed a tent for us, so we slept on a beautiful sandy beach on

Cortes Island where my dad was living. He took me on a walk along the ocean to show me how to find seashells, old pieces of driftwood, plus rocks rounded by the waves on the seashore. We swam in the ocean for the first time and experienced the saltiness on our hair and skin. What fun we had! That same morning my brothers found some juicy peaches on some abandoned trees nearby, and we enjoyed them as snacks all day. I remember the freshness and sweetness of the juice dripping down our faces with every bite.

That day dad and my brother-in-law went looking for a place for us to stay in case of rain. They found a little three-bedroom house on the other side of the island by a beach with egg-sized rocks that roll around when the tide comes in. The house being small and the nights being a bit cold from the tall mountains around, my dad was cutting wood for the stove as he was talking with my mom. I enjoyed watching the love between them. They were so happy to be together again. My dad hadn't shaved, and my mom was red all around her mouth, probably from kissing too much last night. My dad lost his focus and hit his finger with the axe. Red blood was dripping all over and when my mom wiped it, we realized that his finger was cut in half just holding on by the skin. My brother-in-law took him to my cousin's place where they called the hospital, and my dad took his first ride in a helicopter to Campbell River to have his finger stitched. That was scary! My dad couldn't go to work for a while, and we got to spend some time with him.

Our little house had running cold water only and no electricity. My brothers and 2 nephews slept in tents in the yard. My two nieces and I slept in bunk beds on the porch. To go to the bathroom in the middle of the night we had to use a flashlight to find our way to the outhouse. I told my niece that witches lived in the holes, and I got in trouble the next day. Silly teenager.

My brothers and I discovered an old wooden boat situated on the beach close by. The boat must have hit a rock and sunk, then washed up on the beach years ago. We had fun playing pirates. My brothers, nephews and I loved to jump off the large dock and swim around. The ocean was cold and full of harmless jellyfish. The men caught fresh salmon and crabs to cook on the wood stove, and we got our first taste of ocean delicacies.

A small airplane landed on the water once a week to deliver mail to the smallest post office ever (5 x 5 feet). All the kids gathered on the beach to watch the plane take off from the water. Next to the post office was an unclaimed apple tree that we climbed. We ate apples all day long. We got to enjoy adventure better than rich people in a fancy hotel.

We spent a month on the island until school was about to start. We found out that Cortes Island only had a one-room schoolhouse up to grade 6, so we had to move to Powell River because it was the only place that had a school for me and Clement and a boat for dad to ride to work.

Dad clasps my hand warmly and looks into my eyes

shaking me back to the present, "Thank you for the change of scenery. I've enjoyed looking at the beach and the boats."

I am thankful to have the chance to bring a little joy into my mom and dad's life, since they gifted me with a childhood rich with adventure.

When we go home, I help dad out of the car first and take him inside. Then I go back to drag mom out, which is a much bigger job. I must pull her out with both hands, as she is heavy, and take her all the way to the couch and sit her down first before I go back and close the car door.

A few minutes later, the odor in the room changes and I must take mom to the bathroom. I need to undress her and put her in the shower to wash her bottom. It takes a while to clean her, so she slaps my hand as if I am being indecent. My mom's dad was very strict when she was growing up, so she thinks that she must be strict with everyone around her. I just laugh it off. I know she means well and can't express herself anymore.

Between six and seven p.m. the caregiver comes and puts mom's night gown on, but she resists. It is much too early for her since she likes to stay up late at night. She has always been a night owl. My dad is the opposite. He gets up at six o'clock every morning and sit at his desk with his Bible to pray. Raised on the farm, dad woke up early to feed the animals. He likes the freshness and silence of the morning; mom likes the darkness and mystery of the night.

Frank comes back from Vancouver refreshed and

happy, back to being himself again. He gets back into the routine; but when the nurse practitioner comes over, I insist on making sure he gets more respite per week. I want him to have a caregiver babysit my mom and dad in the evening two or three times a week, so he can go out and have some fun. After all, he is single and needs to have a little freedom occasionally. Being on duty 24/7 is a big job for anybody by themselves.

I'm tired and take a break to visit my girlfriend, Claudia. I get a new haircut and a hair peeling on my legs. We go out to the Patricia Movie Theater, buy some popcorn with pop, and go sit ready for a movie. We see Frank walk in, so we invite him to sit with us. We all watch the Walt Disney picture: The Croods. The Powell River theater that was built in 1913 has the original chairs with red-velvet fabric on the seats and ornate carvings on the sides of the wooden armrests.

After the movie, we all go to the pub restaurant across the street. We share some sweet potato fries, drink some herbal iced tea, listen to music and chat. We all go back home refreshed and happy ready to be on duty again.

Points to Remember

Some suggestions to make elders' lives as enjoyable as possible:

Everyone: nurses, doctors, caregivers, family
1) Be gentle, patient, and slow to give elders time to adjust to each situation.
2) Be observant and sensitive to the elders' needs even when they are fussy or picky. There may be a good reason of which you are not aware.
3) Expect the unexpected because elders' inhibitions change.
4) Acknowledge elders as adults even when their behavior is childish, but always protect them if they do something dangerous.
5) Have a sense of humor with mishaps and poor decisions; they are doing the best they can. It's not easy growing old.
6) Consider that elders' perceptions are different from yours because they come from a different generation.
7) Encourage the elders to participate in their own care whenever possible.
8) Be compassionate: their body changes are often causing them pain.
9) Watch for the clues their behavior shows, or simply ask them what they want, whenever possible.
10) Be flexible, and since everyone is different, individualize each situation.

11) Always use your heart with common sense when making decisions for better cooperation.

Family

1) Remember the good times. Happy memories help you through the difficult times.
2) Cherish and be thankful for each moment you have with elders; you never know when it will be their time to go.
3) Spread joy and liveliness: bring a child, dog, cat, or pet to visit elders.
4) Arrange personal grooming since that keeps them more cheerful.
5) Enliven their health with a foot circulation booster machine.
6) Be prepared: get the phone numbers of people that are ready to help in case of an emergency. Make sure you have these numbers easily available for yourself and elder sitters, perhaps on the fridge or a cabinet.
7) Keep the environment clean and organized since it will help make the care easier.
8) Have a washer and dryer handy to help with messes.

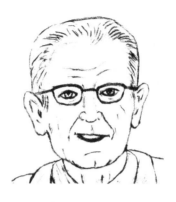

Chapter 4

Dad's Decline and Passing, 2011

Frank calls me: "Dad is in the hospital with pneumonia, and he can't eat anymore!" I book a flight that same night and go to bed. As I close my eyes to go to sleep, I see dad made of light with bright blue eyes. He is standing between two very tall angels made of blue and white light. I feel overwhelmed with tears coming down. I get up, go out of the room so I don't wake my husband up. I'm crying and feel that it is a sign that he will be leaving us very soon! I pray that I get to see him once more before he leaves us.

I'm feeling anxious during the flight: I remember walking through the garden where dad planted roses for my mom. The multicolored rose bushes are enchanting:

the fuchsia-orange roses smell like a mixture of raspberries and rose scent. Some of the bushes have yellow roses, then yellow ones with pink edges, and others that are bright pink. My favorite are the blush-colored large climbing roses by the driveway that smell like paradise. These flowers are the love story of a man that adored his wife and had ten children with her. My father: the romantic, adorable, handsome man who always opened doors for women, helped bring in the groceries, and fixed whatever was broken around the house or yard. He often came in with a rose behind his back with his funny crooked smile to surprise my mom. Then that sweet kiss as he embraced her. He often tickled her, to make us laugh and she'd slapped his hand while giggling.

But times are changing. The two cherry trees don't bear fruit anymore. The plum, apple and pear trees are broken and dried up. The rose bushes are also getting smaller except for the blush climbing roses, vibrating with life, which are bigger every time I come to visit. When I arrive, the gray, sad sky with heavy clouds reflects the mood I'm in. After dinner, Frank drives me to the hospital so we can visit with dad. Frank tells me that he told dad that he can't come home until he can walk by himself. As I peek into dad's hospital room, dad sits up and shout from his bed: "Hi, how are you?"

"Good!" I answer.

"How long are you staying?"

"One month."

"And where are you going to stay?"

"At home with you!"

He says, "Oh I'm so glad!"

He falls back on his pillow, too weak to control his body for very long. I approach him and give him a hug and kiss. I'm so surprised that he recognizes me and that his mind is so clear. His body is frail, just thin skin over his delicate bones; his skeleton face has a yellow tone; his eyes are a bit dry but still blue and recognizable.

The nurses come in with clean sheets to change his bed. They use a sling with pullies to get him off the bed. One of the nurses is young with beautiful long dark hair. He pretends to kiss her and looks at us with that mischievous smile of his. We are all laughing. Frank had teased him a few days earlier about staying in the hospital because he likes the cute nurses. He was returning the joke to make us laugh. His humorous personality is still showing.

The next morning the doctor calls to let us know that there is nothing more that they can do. He says that when the body is shutting down, often the elders get a pneumonia and that it is just a way to help the body let go.

Frank thinks that dad can still start eating again and get better. I call the nurse to see if we can bring him home, but she says no. I talk with her and tell her that I am well educated and so is Clement, who is coming over from the Island today. She gives in, but Frank and I must come at one o'clock to get trained in how to care for him, and he must come home in an ambulance. The nurse also tells us that we must stop the intravenous soon, because it will cause my dad to suffer longer than necessary. His body is shutting down; it's his time to go. Those are the hospital rules, and she advises that we must follow them. We get trained on how to take care of the intravenous, and she gives us many little pink lollipop sponges to dip in water for dad to drink. She tells us that soon we need to detach him from the intravenous because it will cause him to urinate and prolong the suffering.

I hold his hand during the ambulance ride to keep him calm. We put him in the queen-sized bed that he shares with mom. Today his dentures are loose because the bones are deteriorating, so we must take them out. Without his dentures, most of what he says is blurred except for a few simple words or names. He can still say "Frank" and "thank you." "I love you," comes out like clear blue sky.

Frank is exhausted and he goes to sleep downstairs. I'm jetlagged but I must take over. We put mom to bed, and she says: "Who is that man in my bed?" She's feeling uneasy, but I tell her it is dad. I'm too tired to deal with it, so I just go to bed. I get woken up in the middle of the night by noise and voices. I'm so out of it, I take a while to get up. I hear mom complaining. I see my dad trying to hug her or hold her hand, but she smacks him, and I come in just in time. I say, "Mom, it is dad." She moved more to her side of the bed. I go back to sleep then get woken up again. This time I find dad stuck under the closet door still connected to the intravenous, and he is trying to get up. I try to help him up, but I am not strong enough to pull him back on his feet.

Frank had told him that he had to be able to walk before coming home, so he was trying to go to the bathroom on his own. I yell at Frank to run up the stairs and give me a hand. Frank yanks him up and takes him in his arms to the bathroom while I take care of the intravenous carrier and tubes to keep them in one piece and untangled. We both go back to bed but know that we need the hospital bed tomorrow for sure.

I think of mom so scared and upset because she can't recognize dad. I remember as a five-year-old child going to a funeral with my family. It was my mom's uncle in the coffin, and it was scary for me. I realize that now my dad looks just like my mom's uncle. No wonder my mom is freaking out. With her dementia we can't reason with her.

Frank and I decide that we are done with the intravenous, but my sister Frances is coming from Sherbrooke and will be here tomorrow. Frank goes to the pharmacy to buy some Tylenol suppositories for dad's pain. I reconnect the intravenous bottle. When Frank comes back, he scolds me for hooking dad up to the intravenous again. I remind him that Frances wants to see him alive.

He responds, "No, we are done with the intravenous. I can't keep on carrying dad up to the bathroom. It's too much for me; my back is starting to hurt."

My emotions are flying high, and I feel guilty like it is me who is killing him. I go cry in my room and rest. When I come back, I'm a bit better.

Mom won't have anything to do with dad. Frank and I take turns giving dad a drink with the little lollipops. Each time I wet his lips he says: "Thank you. I love you!" and kisses me. Frank manages to convince the hospital that we need the bed immediately even if it is the weekend. Two volunteers arrive and install the bed in the living room. Frank changes dad and puts the pain killer in. Dad fusses a bit, but it works.

I sit by dad's side for a while, but he is asleep now, so I get in bed while I can. I sleep a bit then get woken up by banging noises. I get up and see dad trying to sit up with his hands together in prayer. I sit by his side and sing "Ave Maria" over and over. Dad won't settle down. He starts screaming, "Frank, Frank, Frank!" I get Frank and tell him what I observe. Dad realizes that he is dying, and he is scared. I just can't seem to get him to settle down. Franks says, "I'll get the hymnal of French songs from the special service the church did for mom and dad." He runs downstairs to fetch it. He gives me the booklet, then starts singing the songs and I join in. I learn quickly since I am good at memorizing melodies and follow with the written words. It takes a long time — an hour or two — until dad calms down and falls asleep. We each go back to our rooms and close our eyes for a bit of rest.

The next day Clement arrives and then Patrick. Dad is wide awake and so happy to see them. Patrick picks Frances up from the airport and now there are five of us to take turns. My other brothers Allen and Mike with his wife Patricia come to visit. Then my nephews, some cousins, and some close friends arrive. We all play cards while dad and mom watch us just like we used to in the olden days on Sundays after church. The atmosphere is joyous and fun. We take turns giving dad some water with the sponge. Mom smiles a lot, happy to see us having fun, and dad finally falls asleep.

Frank and I go catch a few hours of sleep while Patrick and Frances take four hour turns sitting beside dad. I take the early morning shift, and then Clement does the next one to let Frank sleep in a bit more. My niece Chrissy and her daughter Shawna bring a French-Canadian Pea soup with bread to share. It is now Sunday March 6th and Frances' birthday is tomorrow. We celebrate her birthday with cake and more card games before everyone leaves for work the next day. Now only Frances, Frank and I remain to share the caregiving, but dad seems asleep all the time, which I think means he is now in a coma.

Monday morning Frances and I go for a walk all the way to Wellington Beach, but we don't talk much. The memories resurface: walking along the beach with dad showings us some seashells and driftwood and telling us stories about the fish he caught, or deer he saw. Coming back, we stop at an antique store nearby, but Frances says, "We better get back home. I have a feeling that dad is ready to go today."

We walk in, have lunch, clean the kitchen, chitchat with Frank and some visitors from church. The minister says a few prayers for my dad. They share a few stories about my dad and then go.

By five o'clock I check on dad and his breath has slowed down a lot. I pray that he waits for me since I go to rest and meditate for a while. When I come back out, Frances and Frank are about to have dinner, but I tell them to turn off the TV and come to dad's side. My sister Frances says, "I'm not hungry anymore." She leaves the hot soup and the bowls on the table.

His breath stops for a few seconds in between each breath. I'm on one side and Frances and Frank are on the other side holding his hand and shoulder. I go close to feel his breath; he does one last long breath on my cheek like his spirit is kissing me on the way out, and he is gone. We take turns calling family members.

I sing the French church songs as the nurse practitioner comes in to make it official. I stop singing, but she asks me to continue, so I do. When I finish the songs, I look at the nurse practitioner, and she has tears rolling down her face. She says, "This is the most beautiful passing I have ever seen. He must have been a very special man. I enjoyed watching you play cards and being so merry." She examines my dad and declares him dead.

We all sit around him and many family members, neighbors, friends come to say their goodbyes. I ask mom if she wants to say "goodbye" to dad, but she says, "No, you go," as she points toward my dad. Frank calls the funeral home and tells them to come at ten o'clock. We have a bit of dinner. We serve coffee, tea, cookies to visitors. We put mom to bed before the funeral home comes to get dad.

Two men dressed in black tuxedos with coattails and white gloves from the funeral home arrive with a rollup bed. They put my dad in a silver-colored bag, zip it up, and take him away. It is official: he is gone and will get incinerated tomorrow. I feel emptiness and a feeling of nausea. I'm so tired, yet so restless and sad.

The next day several family members arrive, even my ex-brother-in-law Renold with his son Ronnie who is my grown-up godson. I haven't seen them in years, and we hug each other with glee. Ronnie still has those big, innocent, brown eyes I love so much. I remind him how he used to put his hands over his eyes when he was upset and run into the wall. He says he still does that, and we laugh. More family and friends arrive, and the house is getting crowded, but I am so happy to see everyone.

I authored a little book about my mom that I read to Shawna, and everyone stops talking to listen tenderly. She is delighted and goes to spend time with my mom, her great grandmother. I watch Shawna sitting on the bed by my mom's side as they look into each other's eyes and smile at each other. Shawna pets her face delicately and tells her she loves her with a kiss on her cheek. Mom is overjoyed with the love and attention. The connection they have is mesmerizing.

We play cards, exchange stories about my dad, and remember the funny jokes he used to tell everyone. Clement says that we can't translate dad's jokes, but I prove him wrong.

I repeat my dad's story (from Chapter 3 about my

grandfather crossing the lake when it isn't frozen enough) to the visitors because they haven't heard it. All our guests are laughing remembering my dad as the great storyteller and jokester.

We take care of the guests while the church members organize a get together for the memorial. They prepare sandwiches, cake, cookies, coffee, tea, and juice in the church basement. The church service is decorated with roses and white lilies. We sing together with all the favorite translations of their regular songs in French: "Amazing Grace (Puissante Grace)", "How Great Thou Art (Son Retour)", "I Surrender All (J'abandonne Tout)". The church members even have somebody film the ceremony for the family in Quebec who can't come to the service.

I wrote a story about my dad when I went to university, and I read it at his Memorial, as follows:

* * *

"There are Things that Money Can't Buy"

"There are things in life that money can't buy -- like joy of life, peace of mind, love and devotion, loyalty, honesty, and integrity, to name a few. This is how I want to introduce my dad to you.

In his youth my dad was a dark blond-haired man with sparkling blue eyes, slanted mischievous smile, dimpled chin, and baby pink skin. He seemed ageless as he played and wrestled with my brothers, worked hard in the garden, and rode his bike five to ten miles a day.

My father had a joy of life or "Joie de Vivre." He always had stories and jokes to tell us at the dinner table each night, and we always had visitors. There were ten of us children and although we had heard most of his stories, thousands of times. We anticipated with laughter the punch line. Like this story: "My dad and his brother were going to pick blueberries. They were surprised to see a bear on the way while they were eating wild cherries. The bear was coming toward them, so they filled their pellet guns with wild cherry seeds. They had the idea to shoot at the bear, which got scared and ran away. The next summer while picking blueberries, they saw a wild cherry tree moving a bit but no wind. What could it be? Then they notice something black moving. Well, it was that some old bear with a cherry tree that had grown on its back." We all burst out laughing because our visitors had believed the story to be true. As it was, most of the story was true except for the ending. Dad got them and the visitors were surprised, and a bit embarrassed but laughing with all of us. It was nice to grow up with so much laughter.

My dad didn't have very many enemies, because when something happened, he was the first one to want to apologize, and work things out. He always wanted to be sure he was being fair and that gave him peace of mind.

I saw love and devotion in my dad often, but what touched me the most was when he got up in the middle of the night to prepare the ice for the hockey games the next day. After the hockey game he would bring both teams home sometimes. My mom received them warmly with coffee, hot chocolate, and cookies.

My father was a gentleman, and the ladies adored him, yet he was loyal to my mother. I remember my mom and dad slowly dancing in the kitchen while the ten of us sat watching at the dinner table. One time the radio was on and the song "Love me tender" by Elvis Presley was on while my dad was eating his dinner. My mom tapped on his shoulder and said, "Papa, papa!" My dad got up and danced with my mom. We all giggled.

I also appreciated my father's honesty. If a cashier made a mistake by giving excess change, he would automatically make it right by giving the right amount of change back.

Another time my mother had just cleaned the kitchen and then left for a couple of hours. When she returned her kitchen was turned upside down. Glass jars and sticky blackberry jam covered the stove and everything else around it! My mother was astonished and asked, "What had happened?" My dad sheepishly admitted that he had cooked some blackberry with a lot of sugar to make some jam. The jam had boiled over. Then he tried putting it in jars but couldn't find the funnel and made a mess. He started to clean up and my mom helped. It took integrity to face the situation.

My dad at seventy-nine years old, still rode his bike five miles a day. In his old age he became too thin, lost a lot of hair, wore dentures, and often talked too much. He was not famous, and didn't have a degree or much money, but there are things in life that money just can't buy."

* * *

We all gather, eat, chat, and remember the good times. We go home to my parents' house where Mom sits in a wheelchair without a clue why there are so many visitors. She enjoys the noise and laughter like old times when we were still living at home, all ten of us. I just can't believe that my dad is gone forever, yet I often feel his presence within me. I am still so much a part of him. I have his artistic, humorous, creative, determined, hard working side that will always live in me. I will forever miss you dad.

Points to Remember

- Remembering the good times helps to soften the sadness of the situation.
- Create the most comfortable situation for the loved one and family.
- Accept the natural emotions that come with the decline and passing of the loved one. Have a cry when you need it, be angry, hit a pillow or yell into the pillow, but if you repress it, you may end up hurting somebody you love with harsh words.
- Go with the flow of events yet stay alert.
- Bring comfort with soft music, singing, and low lighting.
- Take turns with family and friends being with your loved one, day and night so as to not burnout.
- Find information from doctors and nurses about end-of-life signs...
- All these signs together happened in the natural death of my parents:
  o Observe if the patient continues to lose weight, e.g., "down to skin and bones", i.e., can't eat, drink, and walk anymore.
  o The doctor says, "There is nothing else we can do for the patient."
  o The breathing is slowing down and shallow.
  o The skin takes on a lighter glossy, goldish tint.
  o The patient can't wear their dentures, can't swallow, or can't sit up on their own.

o Voice becomes lower and unclear.
o They go into a deep sleep and don't wake up from it (coma).

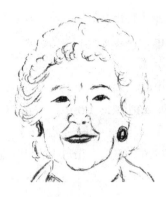

Chapter 5

Mom's Decline and Passing

Mom's mind does not understand that dad is gone forever, but her heart knows, I think because she looks down with a sad pout.

Now that dad is gone, mom has lost her appetite, and she is losing weight.

Occasionally she asks, "Where is dad?"

Sometimes she says, "Dad is at work, right?"

And I say, "Yes!"

I'm not sure what to answer. If I tell her he is dead, she might have a stroke.

I ask Frank what to say, and he tells me that he answers her this way: "Dad is with Jesus."

It is a satisfactory answer for mom; she won't question that. This is less harsh, yet as honest as we can be without upsetting her. The picture of Jesus on the wall reaffirms that, and we keep Mom as peaceful as we can. We invite friends and family to visit, which helps to distract her and get her to eat a bit.

My parents built a large addition to the house twenty years previously, and the Four-Square Church used it for services until they bought a church in Powell River. Sherry, a leader of that church, really appreciates my parents for their contribution. Several years later, Sherry and I became friends when I made a quilt for my parents. Sherry sewed wavy designs on the quilt to finish it for my parents. The quilt has a large farm with a red barn surrounded by animals, pictures of some old antique wringer washers, flowers, and deer. My mom said, "Those are all things from our life!" My parents used the quilt on their queen-sized bed for many years.

Sherry takes me out to a restaurant to eat once a week when I come to help. I don't have a car; therefore, she picks me up each time we go out. My favorite place is in Lund, about twenty miles away from our homestead in downtown Westview. Lund has an old hotel by the ocean with a harbor housing fishing boats, pleasure yachts, sailboats, water taxis, and passenger aluminum boats like the one my dad rode to work some years ago. Just across from Lund, Savary Island has a beige sandy beach that attracts visitors from all over the world. Rumors have it that Elvis Presley and even John Wayne visited it many years ago. Inside the hotel, a couple of little souvenir shops display handmade art: pottery cups, bowls, plates, painted oyster shells and driftwood, and large paintings of sea scenes—sailboats, mermaids, power boats—cover the walls.

She brings me to a little cabin by the sea with outside tables and chairs decked with the charming view of the Lund Harbor, Savary Islands, and the long dock where sea planes arrive to bring the mail and supplies. We can watch the fisher boats bring fresh fish, crabs, and prawns to the shore. The view, soft breeze, and fishy, salty smell of the ocean hypnotize me into a silent appreciation of this perfect sunny, blue-sky day. I eat a couple of homemade tacos with prawns and French fries, a side salad, and sip a cool, icy lemonade. I savor this incredibly fresh food and lovely scenery. I show Sherry the aluminum boat in the harbor below that my dad had to travel to work in from Lund to Teakern Arm. He worked there for so many years before he fell off the boom and the large metal cable fell on his back. He had to retire earlier than planned.

Sherry and I have a lot to share since we both like quilting and love my parents. Over the years, we spend many luncheons eating, talking, and drinking, forgetting about the time. She tells me about the quilt she's working on and invites me to see her work sometime. I share what my parents were like in their younger years. I tell her the story about when I was nine or ten years old one summer. It was raining, and I had nothing to do. I loved drawing people, but I couldn't find any paper or pencils to draw with. I asked Mom if I could draw with white chalk on the living room wall and magically mom said: "Yes!" I chose six record albums from my favorite singers including Ginette Reno, Adamo, Johnny Haliday. I spent the entire day doing their portraits, and mom loved it. When my dad came home from work, he told me, "Erase that. We don't draw on the walls!" My mom came to my rescue and told dad that she didn't want me to erase them. And that was that. The drawings stayed on the wall until they wore off.

My mom understood and supported my artwork and dad's. My dad did hand-carvings when he was younger and in his later years. He used a lathe to shape the wood into bowls, cups, lamps, and other objects. He also made his own knife to shape the wood. Sherry likes the stories I tell her, and I love the stories she shares of her family.

Her daughter and son-in-law are the ministers of the Four-Square Church. They and their two daughters live with Sherry. Sherry's husband helped build a gigantic log cabin-style house with five bedrooms with a very large kitchen giving everyone their own space, but they all ate together. I love the idea of families living in harmony with grandparents. Her husband works out of town, so Sherry would be lonely and feel lost in such a big house if she had lived by herself. I ate with them once and absorbed that lovely warm feeling of togetherness and sharing.

I go back home happy and refreshed each time from our relaxing lunches, like a mini vacation. I am so thankful for my dear friend.

Mom keeps on watching TV but doesn't understand much of it. She eats little and is losing weight. The nurse practitioner takes her off her diabetic and heart pills; they are no longer needed. Frank spends time with her at night and watches old movies or listens to music from her generation. She holds Franks hand tightly and stays awake enjoying old memories.

Tonight, when I put her to bed, I decide to sing the songs she used to sing to us when we were little: "Fait dodo bebe a Maman, fait dodo tu auras du lolo." Which means, "Go to sleep mommy's baby. Go to sleep. I will bring you some water." I sing it a few times then decide to leave her alone, but she either opens her eyes or makes a sound for me to continue. She opens the blanket and pats the bed for me to climb in bed with her, so I do and continue to sing. I whisper another song she used to sing to us from Celine Dion's CD, *Miracle*: "Le loup, la biche et le chevalier. (Une chanson douce)!" She holds my hand for a while until she falls asleep. I feel serene and happy that I can help a bit and give her some joy. The next night I try to do the same, but she pushes me away. She has forgotten about the night before. That is her short-term memory, or else she doesn't need me since her heart is satisfied. I just don't know what to expect; each day is different.

When I need a rest, I walk down to Main Street a few feet down the hill, and visit shops with clothing, yarn, and shoes. My favorite galleries are also close to my parents' house. Powell River is rich with many talented, famous artists: April White who portrays traditional style Native American paintings and Autumn Sky Morrison who creates elaborate spiritual compositions including cosmic scenes and angelic portraits. Luke Raffin does extraordinary realistic paintings of endangered animals in Nature. These artists inspire my artwork at home in Iowa.

Back on duty, I sometimes show mom some picture books: orchids or roses from around the world, fancy teacups with golden brims, flower fairies hidden in nature, babies dressed like flowers! She smiles a lot, squeezes my hand, and says: "I love you," sometimes in words, but more often with closing and opening her eyes, plus moving her lips without sound. We know what she means. It has been her sign to tell us she loves us since we were small. I go home to Iowa happy that I did something to help make her life better.

One Year Later, 2012

Frank calls me: "Mom has been in the hospital with a very bad bladder infection, but she is coming home now."

I book a flight right away, thinking that this must be her time to go. I tell most of this story in Chapter One, but the part I didn't tell the reader is how much I cried as I sat by her bedside. I want to be with mom when she passes, like I did for dad.

It is Norma, the nurse practitioner, who I talk to, and she helps me through my dilemma.

I say, "I want to be with her when she passes away. I don't want her to be alone."

She replies, "Is your mom a very independent women who did things by herself?"

I say, "Yes, she is."

Norma questions me: "Don't you think she wants to go her own way, when she wants to?"

I give in, "I guess so."

"I'm not sure I can come back. My husband hasn't had a nice vacation since I've come to help once a year for the last ten years. He has sacrificed all our vacation money for me to come and help."

Norma explains, "I think she wants to die alone. You need to let her do it her way."

My heart is hurting, I cry and cry, my eyes are all puffy and red, my hair is messy. I just can't resign myself to not being here by my mom's side. I decide to go out to dinner at the Asian restaurant by the ferry boat just down the street. I sit outside at a table looking at the ocean. I am feeling sad, not sure that I can come back to be with mom next time. I see a lady sitting at the table next to me. We are both alone eating our dinner. The air is fresh with a soft breeze. The sun is still bright, and the ocean is a dark blue.

I look at the lady at the next table who greets me and explains that she is in Powell River on business. I tell her I came to help take care of my mom, but I am going home tomorrow. I disclose my secret that I am upset because I don't think I can afford to come back next time to be with my mom for her last days.

She frowns, "Oh, I am so sorry."

We are silent for a while and suddenly she exclaims: "Look over there, It's a mother whale with her baby in the ocean!"

I turn my head and discover the big orca whale's back and her large fin sticking out with her baby tagging along on her side. All at once, they both shoot water through their blowholes. I am ecstatic; I can't believe my luck. Orca whales don't usually come this close to the city. I feel it is a sign that I will be back next year, but I am not sure how. This gives me hope that something good will happen. I leave feeling better that somehow everything will be all right.

Trip Back

Next year Frank calls, and again I think it is mom's time to go. We can't afford the plane ticket, but my husband, Ron, says: "Go, we will put it on the credit card and somehow it will all work out." On the way in the airplane, I think of my mother-in-law who had Alzheimer's. We saw her two days before she passed. She was in a coma. I remembered how she prayed the rosary every morning and every night, so I decided to say some "Hail Mary's!" While sitting beside her, she suddenly moved her mouth with the prayer as I was saying it. Somehow the memories of the prayer seemed to help. I hope it gave her some comfort.

I arrive back and mom is sleeping. She wakes up, happy to see me. She squeezes my hand, and I kiss her tenderly. She looks almost lifeless, but her eyes follow me where I come and go. I sit beside her just to feel her presence with me. It is so hard to think she won't always be there and that I will have to let her go.

I had written an email to Norma, the nurse practitioner, but she says that she has a new boss that won't let me visit at her monthly staff meeting. She wanted me to tell the story of all the changes I did the last time I was here. Norma was impressed with the changes in routine that I made for the caregivers. I found a way to communicate with mom using some cards with notes on them that mom can read. The notes are written big and in French with English at the bottom for the caregivers as you may remember from the first chapter.

I get up early and go to the glass doors to look at the ocean and enjoy the early pastel-colored sunrise. I check on mom. I put a chair by her bed, hold her hand, and do my quiet meditation. I peek to see how she is doing, and I see her facial expressions soften and relax. Meditation has as good effect on her as it does on me. The next morning when I go to her bedside, she is awake and points to the chair and the bed. I bring the chair by her bed and meditate with her again. With her dementia I wonder why she remembered what I did yesterday? Her facial expressions relax, and we enjoy a special deep silence together.

The days are long and boring, so I try to find more things to do with mom. I show her the booklet I wrote about her with some of the stories about advice she gave us. I read it to her. She smiles with an expression of approval, shaking her head up and down with a "yes". Mom and I share birthdays. Hers is the 28th of November and mine is the 26th. On my birthday my daughter, who was mad at me before, calls to wish me a happy birthday. After the call, I am crying because our relationship has been so hard. My mom grabs my hand and gently pulls me towards her. I put my head on her chest and cry, she pats my back just like she used to. For that moment, I have my mom back, but then she pushes me away, points to my room and says: "Go to bed." She is still the same mom I know even if she is frail and weak. Her personality is still there. I go to my room and rest for a while.

Mom sleeps a lot but stays awake when we have visitors. Her friend Jean that she hasn't seen for many years comes to visit, but mom doesn't recognize her at all. Jean colors her nails, yet mom doesn't respond much. Is she mad at Jean or does she not recognize her? We just don't know.

It is time for me to go home. My daughter is getting married in a few days, so I come to say "goodbye" to mom. Mom starts talking, saying: "The doctors… hospital… hurt." I get worried and have a hard time leaving but must catch that plane to Vancouver, so I run out. I feel bad but I can't stay.

I get in a small airplane from Powell River, and we take off. We go through a storm cloud and the airplane is shaking with loud cracking sounds. I feel like I'm in a tin can about to crash, but within 10 or 15 minutes we come out of the cloud and land at the Vancouver airport with no problem, safe and sound.

I get Patrick to call Frank when I arrive in Vancouver.

I want to know how mom is doing. Frank says that mom is fine; she just didn't want me to go and was trying to manipulate me.

On the way home I think of my uncle, my dad's oldest brother, who loved fishing. He lived in my parents' basement suite. The fan over his stove was directly over my parents' fan. Every time my uncle cooked some bizarre fish that he had caught, we would get the awful smell upstairs. Uncle went fishing every day when it was nice out, and we never knew what he would bring home. He didn't have a sense of smell anymore and probably not much taste left either. Everyone at the house would complain about the distasteful smells. Being in his eighties, he had the bad habit of standing in his boat when he caught a fish. He fell in a few times and got rescued. The police brought him back one day very mad at my parents for letting him go by himself. They threatened and ordered my parents to keep him home, or else.

I came to visit my parents with my two small children one morning decades ago since I only lived a mile away. I saw my old uncle unshaved, with dirty clothes on, looking down at the floor, and not responding when I greeted him. I asked mom and dad what was the matter and was he sick? Mom explained to me that she and dad wouldn't allow uncle to go fishing because the police threatened them. I said, "He looks like he is going to die of sorrow." Mom and dad gave up and let uncle go fishing on his own again. A few years later after I moved to Iowa, I called home to say "hello!" My sister Barb answered the phone and told me: "There was a storm that came up in early evening and uncle wasn't back from fishing. We called the Coast Guard. They shot some rescue flares in the sky. We were watching through the glass doors. They found uncle under his boat floating face down. It looked like fireworks in the sky celebrating uncle's life! He died happy doing what he wanted to do."

My plane stops in Denver, but the next plane is overcrowded, so no room for four people and one of them is me. The agent offers $400.00 for anybody who gives their seat up and flies later. Three people give up their seats for one who is pregnant, another who is going to a funeral and the other, a crippled elder in a wheelchair. I'm the only one without a seat. The next plane to Cedar Rapids is in 6 hours, but I see that there are planes that go to Des Moines every hour. I ask the agent at the desk if I could take an airplane to Des Moines instead because I don't want to wait 6 hours, since my husband and grandson are on their way to the airport already. She says that United Airline will reimburse my ticket for that. It is their policy. I figure that she means just my ticket from Denver to Iowa. The manager calls me and gives me a $1,250.00 check and a new ticket for Des Moines. I am shocked but very happy. This is the cost of my ticket for my whole trip that is on our credit card. I just can't believe it. My belief is confirmed: when you do a good deed, some good comes back to you. Now I must reach my husband and tell him to switch airports and drive another two hours, but I tell him about the money first. Renny is happy the ticket money pays the full price of the credit card. It's the fourth of July, so we see the fireworks on the way home from the different cities along the highway.

A year later, 2014

Frank calls to tell me that mom hasn't been eating for eight days now. It is my daughter's birthday, so I tell her to come over to my house with her four children to say their goodbyes to their grandmother. Renny connects the computer to the TV to communicate and see my mom for a visit. Mom is skin and bones. Her face is bloodless white with a yellow tone. I know it is the end for sure this time. I introduce each great grandchild and my daughter Mel's husband who she hasn't met. We tell her we love her and send her kisses. Mel says, "Sing some songs for her." I chorus "Son Retour" ("How Great Thou Art"). The blanket is moving so Frank checks it out and pulls mom's hand out. She is waving back at us. I just can't believe it. She's about to die and she is waving at us. We say our goodbyes, shut off the TV, and have a cry.

The next night I still go to my writing class and write about letting mom go. I come home and decide to go to sleep. I hear the phone at twelve-fifteen, and it is Frank. Mom passed away around 10 o'clock which is twelve o'clock in Iowa. I cry and have a hard time going back to sleep.

The church organizes a memorial for my mom and my brother Patrick connects me with his laptop. I send money to Sherry for two dozen multi-colored roses and Patrick buys two dozen white roses. The songs are the same as my dad's memorial except for the song my mom used to sing: "Les Roses Blanches" ("The White Roses"). The song tells a story about a little boy whose mom is sick. He steals some white roses to bring to his mom because she loved them so. The church looks beautiful, and I get to read a poem for my mom. Everyone comes to say "hi" after the service. I have been there with mom in spirit the whole time, so she didn't really die alone after all.

I am so thankful for all the church members' help.

My Fondest Memories of Time with Mom

I remember sleeping outside on the balcony at our old house on the hill by the highway in Quebec. The balcony had no railing, so mom had to supervise us because it was the flat roof of the room they added to the downstairs. Mom got us to dress in our pajamas, bring some comforters with pillows, and we had a Saturday night sleep out. Lightning bugs lit up the dark, clear sky revealing a view of the lake. A soft breeze tickling our faces. It wasn't too hot or cold, just perfect weather. Mom made a huge bowl of popcorn for all of us: me, a 10-year-old, and my younger brothers Patrick and Frank, six and five, with my sister's stepchildren Francis and Bob, also six and five, plus sweet four-year-old Sasha. Mom was showing us that the pieces of popcorn have shapes that sometimes resemble animals' heads. We ate popcorn, told some silly jokes, then mom sang us some songs to put us to sleep. I was older, so I didn't fall asleep for a while, and I watched the stars and moon come out. It was a magical night, and we had a good time with mom. Mom was usually too busy with chores to be with us, so it was a very special treat to have her full attention that night. In the morning, she made a large stack of buckwheat pancakes with butter and maple syrup, a delightful French-Canadian tradition. My brothers and nephews competed to see who could eat the most pancakes, which kept mom busy making more pancakes all morning.

I often think of the times she let me cry in her arms and soothed me with comforting words. I still feel her hugs, especially when I wear her nightgown that I kept and cherish. I am thankful that she stayed home as much as she could. I loved the Christmases, Easters, and birthdays I celebrated with her. Her nourishing qualities and wise advice helped me through the years: "put yourself in the other person's shoes; time arranges things; put your sorrows in God's hands; if a man truly loves you, he will love your children."

When I was eleven, we moved to the newer house down the hill away from the highway. My dad had bought a house and had big trucks move it there for my mom. When winter came, I needed a hat. Mom had yarn that changed colors from beige to an orange-red. She surprised me after school with a beautiful French beret she knitted for me. I was amazed since I didn't know she could knit. I wore that beret stylishly like mom had shown me everywhere I went. I cherished that hat for many years to come. My teens years were difficult because my sister, now married, had taken care of me most of my life. My mom didn't know me very well and didn't understand me, but in her old age she learned to appreciate my sensitivity and caring abilities. Love you mom, and I miss you every day.

Points to Remember

1) Bring peace, love, and joy when you can.
2) Be grateful for the love and help that friends and family give you!
3) Do good, believe in goodness, and good will come back to you.
4) Good intentions and deeds get rewarded by the Almighty, Nature, God, or Angels, whichever you believe in.
5) Use new technology to be with your loved one when you can't be there physically.
6) Be there in spirit if you can't be there at all.
7) Do what you can and don't have regrets.
8) Celebrate your loved one's life and the memories you have built together.
9) Cherish your final moments together.
10) Let your loved one go the way they want to leave this world.
11) Memorials are so much more enjoyable than funerals.
12) Cherish the qualities inherited from your parents and love yourself for it.
13) Keep the good and let go of the bad.

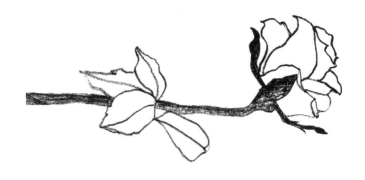

Chapter 6

Self-Care for Caregivers

Caregivers' burnout is very common.

Caregiving is an especially important task that is easier for you if you are at your best.

In earlier chapters I tell you the breaks I took, but there is more to it than that.

"Being well" means physically, emotionally, spiritually, and intellectually.

Here are some suggestions to keep well:

For the body

- Good sleep each night with a routine that works for you.
- Good healthy food (fresh and organic) if possible.
- Daily multi vitamins with vitamin D3 and calcium for bones.

- Oil treatments with body massages that are refreshing and rejuvenating.
- Bubble baths with a soothing scent, essential oils like rose, lavender or others you may like.
- Exercises or sports every day.
- A walk after dinner.

For the mind and heart
- Go out for fresh air and sunshine.
- Listen to soft music.
- Enjoy some silence, meditation, or prayers.
- Have some fun and adventures on your days off.
- Talk with friends.
- Spend time with positive family members.
- Visit a museum.
- Attend a lecture.
- Read a book.

For outside support
- Schedule others to take over for you periodically to give you respite from caregiving.
- Regular visits to the doctor to keep well.
- Going to your physiotherapist or chiropractor (especially if you must do some lifting) to keep your spine and bones healthy.
- Consider counseling for professional advice and support.

Nourish yourself to live happier each day. Good moods are contagious!

The better you feel, the better you respond to crisis.

About the Author

Roseline Woods was born in a little village near Sherbrooke, Quebec, Canada, speaking French.

She is the eighth child of a family of ten children. One of her oldest sisters, Frances, was very studious and an excellent artist. Frances would allow Roseline to sit by her side when she did homework and give her colored pencils and paper. Frances taught her the alphabet and sometimes read to her. This is how Roseline found support for her drawings and discovered her love of writing.

Roseline loved to write about the beauty of her surroundings. At the age of fourteen, her sister got married and Roseline missed her. The family moved to the province of British Colombia about two hundred miles north of Vancouver where her dad had found work. She had to learn English and adjust to the environment which delayed her writing.

She had three children from two previous marriages.

For twelve years she ended up raising her children by herself. For the past twenty-two years she has been happily married to a man that loves her children.

When her son turned eighteen and she turned forty, she decided to go to university. She received a B.A. in Art and Elementary Education. Her thinking was still in French, so she had to do several classes in English to upgrade her ability to do her assignments. This is when she found her love of writing again. After helping take care of her grandchildren and her parents, she finally found the time to write. She now has a lot of experiences in caregiving and a full heart, so she decided to write this book.

About The Illustrator

Roseline's ability to draw came at an early age and her favorite was to draw people.

At four years old she drew her version of Donald Duck dancing the twist. When she was ten years old, looking and not finding pencils or paper, she asked her mom if she could draw on the wall with chalk. Her mom gave her permission. She drew six faces of her favorite French singers of that time; Adamo, Ginette Reno, Johnny Haliday to name a few. In her school she was known as being the best artist in the whole school. When her youngest daughter was nine years old, Roseline did a BA in Art and realized her dream, but family duties took her in a different direction for a while.

Roseline remarried in 2000. Her husband and she helped her oldest daughter and did what they could in helping with four grandchildren. Roseline took care of her health first then went to study portraiture and more with Mary Muller in Des Moines, Iowa. She has done over 200 classes with Mary. She has exhibited her work in several galleries and has done the cover painting and all illustrations in this book.

Printed in the USA
CPSIA information can be obtained
at www.ICGtesting.com
LVHW050749171023
761311LV00003B/17